Self-Care Basics For Helping Professionals

Jennifer Millette

DEDICATION

This book is dedicated to all of the helping professionals I have known and worked with through the years. You have all taught me so much and inspired me in numerous ways.   I also dedicate this book to those unfortunate cashiers I wasn't always as nice to as I should have been. Thank you for your patience on my bad days, though that's never an excuse. I promise, I'm getting better and being kinder, though am still a work in progress.

CONTENTS

ACKNOWLEDGMENTS

Thanks to Tina Diel for being both my model and second photographer in the book, and to Anna Castle for generously letting us use her beautiful studio, Yoga Castle, for one of our photo shoots. Thanks also to my Cortiva Institute classmates and faculty for participating in our yoga classes at school. Finally, thanks to my teacher Ken, who asked me the greatest question when I'd been doubting my abilities: "Why did you think that?" I had no response, and therefore no excuse.

1 INTRODUCTION

As I sit here working on this book's final edit, I'm also enjoying a new coffee shop. In fact, this place is so cozy that it inspired me to stay longer, go back out to my car, grab these pages and dive in. Strange as that may sound, this is part of my self-care plan.

See, I write because I enjoy it, and I feel compelled to share this information with others. I get in a zone, in flow as they say, and savor the creative aspect of it. If it ever feels like work, I stop right then and there. It won't serve me at that point, or you as the reader. Of course, I have the luxury of not relying on my writing for a paycheck. Leaving one's paying day or main job because it's not fun anymore might not be an immediate option for most. But as a recovering workaholic, I am all too familiar with the tendency to push through when I'm miserable. I counter those former habits by recognizing unnecessary 'work', and making another, healthier, and more enjoyable choice whenever possible. Today I'd already worked a long shift at the above referenced day job. The last thing I felt like doing at this point was something effortful like editing, even though it had seemed like a good idea this morning. So, physically weary and mentally drained, I gave myself permission to change the plan. I decided to still go the coffee shop-something I'd been looking forward to for a few days-but let it truly be just a treat- a delicious beverage and some seated rest time. I deliberately left the book pages in the car so they couldn't guilt me into looking at them "for just a minute or so". Free of that self-induced pressure, though, something interesting happened.... I ended up inspired and remembered that writing-and sometimes even editing-is fun for me. So, I got the pages, read through and did some leisurely rewrites, all the while taking time to enjoy my coffee, look around, breathe slowly and savor being in this new place. I was inspired because I gave myself the free space to become so. And really, that's what self-care is all about. Giving yourself space to figure out what you need, giving it to yourself, and savoring the results.

The original impulse to write this book came from my experiences during my time in massage therapy school and afterwards as a new massage therapist. Before then I'd been specifically in the health and wellness industry for about 10 years. One of the perks of being a full-time yoga and Pilates instructor was being healthy and fit. When I changed careers, however, I realized I'd severely overestimated my ability and willingness to keep the level of health and fitness that came from teaching multiple classes a day. Who has that kind of time? But as I looked closer, I had to admit that what was happening-weight gain, sluggishness, achy joints and soreness beyond the physical rigors of massage-were due to some pretty mindless choices on my part. Even though I knew better, I'd gotten pulled into the culture of vending machines, fast food lunches and community donuts. I was also getting swept up in old tendencies to react instead of respond, get too focused on the details and stress over the small stuff. At the same time, I had met such wonderful people and wanted to somehow give something back. I also needed to make myself accountable and start practicing the things that I knew would help improve my health and fitness, lower my stress, and keep my life more in balance.

As I started to write this book, however, I thought back on all the different places I've worked and different jobs I've had through the years. I've done everything from social work to retail, to bartending and serving. All these jobs have been working directly with people in some type of service role. Most places I've worked have had the telltale break room with florescent lights and no windows. But all of them had people there who truly wanted to help others, who meant well and really cared about their jobs. People who deserved to be happy and healthy. I also realized that in all those places, I'd ended up focusing much of the time on helping those fellow employees manage stress in some form or another. A lot of my passion for subsequently teaching yoga, meditation and Ayurveda came from inspiring people to go out there and do their job from a place of inspiration, enthusiasm and just feeling good. So, I decided to rewrite the book with a new, expanded focus to include all helping professionals.

I define that as anybody on the front lines of somehow providing service to or interacting with the public for their job.

 I chose the practices in this book because they've made a huge impact in my life, and they are efficient and effective in promoting overall health and happiness. The information provided here is shared with the understanding that each reader's situation is unique. There is no single right way to incorporate these into your life. Self-care, by definition, is all about the self. It becomes whatever you need it to be.

So, if you are reading these pages, congratulations. it means that you've decided to make yourself a priority in your life. You deserve this. When you take time for yourself, everybody benefits, in all areas of your life. Doing this won't always be easy, but I promise you that it will always be worth it. Thank you for allowing me to join you on this journey and be open to the possibilities. Maybe together, we can rethink and restructure the workplace, so that the ideas and practices shared in this book are automatically built into all places of employment. One breath at a time.

Peace, love and radiance,

Jen

2 SELF-CARE: WHO CARES?

Self-care is pretty much what it sounds like-actions intended to take care of yourself. This phrase tends to be used in context of an environment where the act of self-care involves deliberate actions, choices and separate time away from or carved out of a schedule.

For many, self-care sounds like a luxury, a treat, something at the bottom of your to-do list, if it even made the list in the first place. It's generally not given a lot of time or attention. It becomes the thing that will happen later, except later never comes. There's not a lot of value placed on it. It's far more acceptable-even encouraged-to just tough things out rather than take time to replenish and restore. Which is interesting, considering that athletes actually get stronger on their rest days. Some mistakenly consider taking time for themselves a sign of weakness or incompetence. It's safe to guess that many people don't really prioritize, or even care about self-care.

Yet we should. For many reasons.

Looking back, I now realize that I wasn't doing the world any favors when I was out there as an overworked, multi-tasking stress monster (hence my dedication at the beginning of the book to the poor cashiers who had to deal with me in that state). Energy is contagious, so I was most likely spreading my stress wherever I went. This also affected the quality of my work, my relationships and my health. Research backs this up...stress related illnesses can result in lowered work productivity and increased revenue loss due to sick days. At this point, virtually all illness can in some form be linked back to stress. Quite frankly, stress can make you miserable, affecting both your physical and mental health. The good news is that no matter your individual situation, you have a lot of control over how you take care of yourself and manage your stress. This is where your self-care practice comes into play.

3 THE WHY OF WORK: HOW TO USE THIS BOOK

While self-care is important for everybody, I've focused on the world of work because, quite frankly, this is the easiest place to find you. This is where so many of us spend the bulk of our time, whether in an actual physical workspace, logging flexible hours from home, or using your so-called free time checking emails, completing work tasks or worrying about work related matters. Our self-concept and identity are formed largely based on our choice of job or career. This includes those who may work within their own home as the family house manager and/or caretaker.... except they don't get the benefit of a paid salary and are literally at work the minute they wake up in the morning! Work is a primary source of our stressors, whether it's about the time spent at or traveling for work, the personalities we must deal with, the amount of money we are/aren't paid for our labors, or the work tasks themselves. Helping professionals are prone to this, as so much of their time is spent dealing with others, anticipating their needs and problem solving if those needs can't be realistically met.

Finally, for some (me included), work becomes an excuse, a place to hide, or even an addiction. Releasing its vice grip on us can lead to more enjoyment of actual time spent on the job, as well as improvements in other areas of our lives.

The reasons for working in a job or field vary. Some do it because it's their passion, what they feel they were born to do. Others chose it for other factors like salary, location, benefits, etc. Still others chose it because it may bridge a financial gap, help fund a specific goal, or maybe it was the only job they could find that matched their qualifications.

The reasons you're in your current job or field affect how you feel about it, your experience when you're there, and the kind of self-care choices that will benefit you the most. This book offers several different types of these. Specifically, information about meditation, yoga and Ayurveda will be shared. These practices have made a huge impact in my life. They are efficient and effective in promoting overall health, happiness in all areas. Some of the specific strategies may click with you right away, others not so much. My intention in writing this book is for you to take what you need from it. Whether that's a single technique listed, a handful of your favorites, or just make a general commitment to actually taking time for yourself. You control this, so design it however works best for you.

4 MEDITATION

The ancient practice of meditation is getting a lot of attention these days. Meditation is basically flexibility work for the mind. It increases the ability to relax as well as to focus. By practicing meditation, one learns how to notice things that are occurring without being distracted by them. This first lowers the volume of the thoughts in our minds, then slows them down.

Our current lifestyles have left stress running rampant. Negative emotions like irritation, anxiety or anger release stress hormones in our bodies, which contributes to toxicity. Meditation is an antidote to this stress response by helping reduce its negative effects on the body. Research now shows that regular meditation practice can lower blood pressure, strengthen the immune system, and decrease fatigue. In fact, the American Heart Association has endorsed Transcendental Meditation (known as TM) as a complementary therapy for lowering blood pressure. Meditating on a regular basis also leads to more energy, better sleep, improved vitality and focus. These effects, not surprisingly, help you become more pleasant to be around and therefore improve your interpersonal relationships.

At work, meditation benefits can mean fewer sick days, more effective and efficient work, and getting along better with peers, clients and supervisors. Even if nothing else about your workplace changes, this single change that you make for yourself can have a significant, lasting impact on your work experience, and well being in general. For me, meditation was the self-care tool that most impacted my life, which is why it's the first technique I discuss here.

HOW TO MEDITATE

For all its benefits, starting a meditation practice can seem daunting in today's world. We are expected to constantly be doing several things at once throughout our day, so the idea of sitting and focusing on one thing can seem very difficult and looked down on. Our brain naturally wants to rebel and keep itself busy. Finding time for one more thing to do can feel overwhelming. This can be understandably discouraging when trying to learn how to meditate. One of the most frequent concerns new meditators have is not being able to get their mind to turn off. This is because there's a popular misconception that meditation is supposed to make your mind completely still. This is unrealistic. The mind is designed to think, and it's going to keep thinking! Thoughts are naturally occurring events, if we don't perseverate on them and let them take over. In fact, to let your thoughts occur without paying much attention to them cleanses your mind. So don't try to force your mind to stop thinking-this creates resistance both in the mind and in the body. Instead, imagine your thoughts just floating in and out of the sky of your mind, like clouds on a summer day. Before long you will find your mind starting to slow its roll a bit, or even more.

To set yourself up for success, it's important to have a place, a plan, and strategies to use during practice. Choose a location where you can regularly meditate at home, as well as a possible second one for times at work when you need to recharge or calm down. It should be a place where there will be minimal interruptions with relative quiet. At work, I have sometimes gone to meditate in my car, or gone for a mindful walk if needed. There are no hard and fast rules to choosing your regular meditation space. It should feel safe and peaceful, with minimum distracting clutter. You may choose to have a few inspiring mementos close by, use relaxing scents like vanilla or lavender, or play instrumental music or nature sounds, but none of these are required in order to meditate.

For best results, meditate every day. Not only will this help it become a regular habit (especially if you link it with another habit like brushing your teeth), but it will make the results more powerful in a shorter amount of time. Ideally it should happen in the morning at the start of your day, so your mind isn't distracted by thoughts of your day already in progress. At least 5 minutes a day is a good start, working your way up to 15-20 minutes. The following picture is a common seated posture, a yoga pose called Easy Pose, often used for meditation. You can also sit in a chair with feet on the floor if that is more comfortable, or if you're doing a short mini meditation at your desk at work, or in your car on break.

Easy Pose

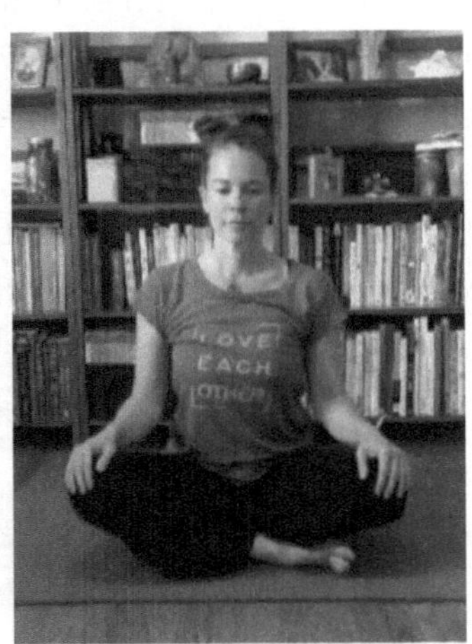

- *Sit on mat, pillow, blanket or bolster.*
- *Inhale, bend knees and cross ankles.*
- *Exhale, draw navel into spine.*

MEDITATION TECHNIQUES

Depending on where and how you plan to meditate, techniques can range from more passive, where you listen to somebody or something, to more active, such as focusing on a specific word, phrase or sound. Most styles require little, if any props, other than yourself and a willingness to try something that might not feel natural or comfortable at first. It may take some time, but it's worth it.

Progressive Muscle Relaxation

This can be practiced as a technique on its own, or before doing another meditation. The goal is to relax the body, one section at a time. The action of contracting, then releasing each part helps remind the muscles to return to their natural relaxed state, rather than remain in the state of tension that they might be holding onto out of habit. You can do this seated or lying down. Starting with the tips of the toes and working up to the crown of the head, squeeze muscles tight for a count of 3, then release them. Do this in sections: first with feet and toes, then legs and glutes, then torso, then fingers and hands, then arms and shoulders, then face, then finally the entire body.

Guided Meditation/Visualization

This type of meditation involves listening, either seated or comfortably reclined, to a speaker guide you through meditation by reading a script specifically designed to relax you and slow the mind. This can be done in person, or through listening to audio or video recordings. Guided meditations can be considered a complete practice on their own. They are also a common form of meditation used at the end of a yoga practice or class during relaxation.

Guided meditations can have specific topics such as self-esteem, empowerment, physical strength, increased focus, powerful leadership or professional success. They may also promote physical healing, from injury or illness, or facilitate pain management. The possibilities are endless. Regardless of intention, they usually start by focusing on the breath and body, then shift to a visualization (i.e., mountains, clouds, trees or the ocean) designed to take you to deeper levels of relaxation. While in this deeper relaxed state, your subconscious is open to positive suggestions. Afterwards, you will be slowly guided back to your normal state of awareness, leaving you feeling refreshed. A guided meditation can last anywhere from 5 minutes to an hour, though a meditation session of 15 minutes or longer is recommended to maximize the benefits.

Mindfulness

A popular concept associated with meditation is mindfulness. Mindfulness literally means to let your mind become full of whatever is happening now, in the present moment. When your mind is present, it's not replaying the past or worrying about the future. Mindfulness is not a relaxation technique, as you are actually increasing focus of the conscious mind, but the fact that it pulls the mind out of the past and future does create a peaceful, yet alert effect. This seems to be a less intimidating approach for many would-be meditators than the traditional idea of completely stopping the mind, which can seem overwhelming in today's plugged in, multi-tasking world. Despite feeling like they have too much on their minds at any given point in time, most people are mindless as they go about their day. They're physically there, but not truly there. Their mind is caught in their anger, their regrets, worries, and fears, instead of focused in their body. You are caught in the past or in the future, places that don't exist because they have already occurred or might occur (or not!) later.

On the other hand, mindfulness occurs when the body and mind are in the same place, having the same experience. When your mind is there with your body, you are established in the present moment. It's in that real, true moment that you can tap into the natural state of peace that already exists within you.

Mindfulness can be applied to any daily activity, whether it is driving to work in the morning, taking a walk around the neighborhood, or preparing dinner for the family. Meditations exist for washing dishes and making yourself a cup of tea! Just about anything you do, you can do it mindfully.

Mindfulness practices are just completely noticing what's happening, not furrowed concentration or effort. They should be as effortless and natural as the flow of breath itself. At first, however, it can feel strange because you're not used to that steady, level focused feeling in your mind. In fact, your mind may try to resist this by going back to its old habits of running back to the past or future, where it can comfortably get irritated or anxious, like its used to doing. To help minimize your mind going rogue, imagine instead that you are watching yourself from a distance, going about your daily activities. If excessively distracting thoughts continue to creep in, change the thought simply by thinking "I am…." And then complete the sentence with whatever activity you happen to be doing at that exact moment. (again, this works even when washing the dishes!). Continue to silently repeat that thought, so that other thoughts get crowded out.

Mindful Breath Meditation

Mindful breathing is one of the most common mindfulness techniques. As well as all the other benefits of meditation already listed, additional benefits of mindful breath meditation include enhanced lung capacity and breath efficiency.

Sit up tall. As you inhale, think "Inhaling in". As you exhale, think "Exhaling out". Continue thinking "Inhaling in" on your inhale, and "Exhaling out" on your exhale. Allow for slight, natural pauses when you are finished inhaling and exhaling, so you aren't rushing the breath. Your mind might start to slow a bit. If your thoughts start to wander to other topics, just gently guide your mind back to your breath, silently repeating "Inhaling in…. Exhaling out…." Continue for 1-5 minutes.

Walking Meditation

Literally take steps forward in your life while remaining fully present in the moment. No additional physical effort beyond the act of walking is needed. Allow the breath to sync up with your steps by allowing the inhale to last a certain number of steps (whatever is comfortable for you), and the exhale lasting the same number of steps. Think something along the lines of "I am walking…..I am stepping my right foot forward….now my left foot forward….". You get the idea. This rhythmic quality to your synced-up steps, combined with the attention on both moving body and flowing breath, create a powerful meditative experience.

Meditation With Affirmations or Intentions

Using specific affirmations or intentions during meditation plants the seed in the subconscious mind and increases the chance that they will eventually materialize in real life. This is due to you becoming more open to their possibilities, alert to opportunities about the topic that may show up, and starting to act in ways that support the goal coming to fruition.

Find your comfortable meditation posture. Notice the breath, hearing and feeling the inhales and exhales throughout your body. Silently repeat your chosen, present tense ("I am...") intention or affirmation (See samples below if you are looking for ideas). Keep repeating this at a slow, relaxed pace. Let the breath naturally flow, silently repeating the phrase at a rhythm that feels natural for you. Whenever your mind wanders-and it will, but that's normal, so it's ok-, just guide it back to the breath, then your affirmation. Meditate for up to 15-20 minutes if possible.

Here are some sample affirmations you might use:

- I am calm
- I am strong
- I am enough
- I inhale peace.... I exhale love
- I inhale love...I exhale tension
- I inhale faith.... I exhale fear

Meditation Apps

There are several mediation apps available today that will guide you through the above meditations. These include Calm, Mindful, and Headspace. Some of them also have features that log your previous meditations so you can keep track of your progress. You can also find audio recordings of guided visualizations on iTunes.

MUDRAS

Mudras have been called yoga poses for the hands. They direct the body's energy, called prana, with specific intentions behind them that can promote specific effects. They can be used during meditation or done on their own.

Energy Charger

Place palms together in front of heart center. Rub together until warm, then take slightly apart to feel energy pulsing between them. Promotes energy, empowerment and focus. Option to place warm hands over closed eyes (not pictured) if dealing with vision fatigue (computer screens, etc.) or a headache.

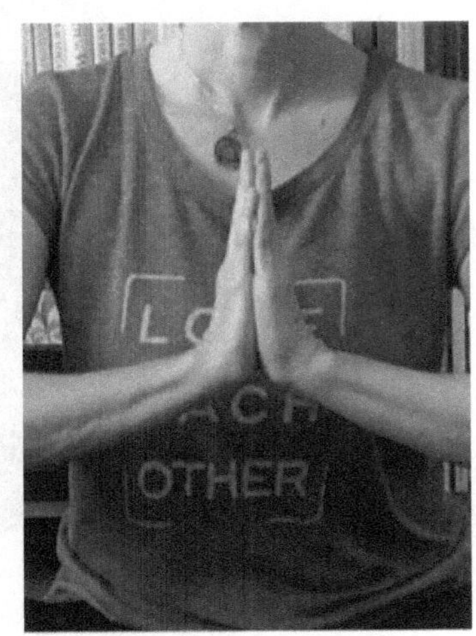

Lotus Mudra

The lotus is a widely recognized symbol in yoga. This flower that grows in mud acknowledges humble beginnings, and celebrates that we are the culmination of all our life experiences, both positive and challenging, up to the present moment.

Take hands together at heart, palms together. Keep thumbs and pinkies together, open the palms into a lotus shape. Focuses the mind, opens the heart, promotes feeling connected to others.

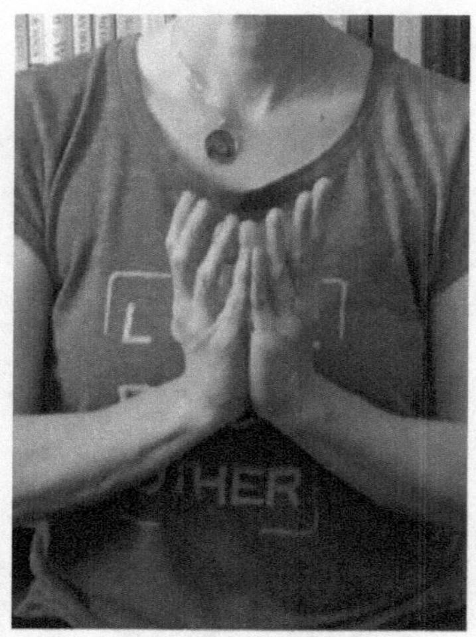

Wisdom Mudra

Make the 'ok' sign with each hand, tips of index fingers and thumbs to touch. rest hands on thighs or let arms rest next to sides. Alleviates anxiety, quiets the mind, increases lung capacity.

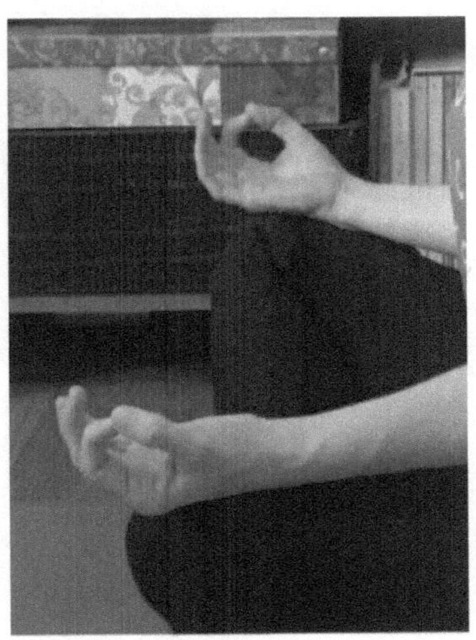

Some effects of your meditation practice you'll notice right away. You'll start to remember how it feels to not be in a constant state of go, go, go. You'll become more consciously aware of your breathing, even outside of your dedicated meditation times. Over time, you'll start to use mindful breathing and affirmations as strategies during stressful experiences, and before challenging situations where you know you need to be very present and focused on others. You may even catch yourself becoming less frustrated in traffic! (A great place to practice mindful breathing, by the way). Eventually you'll start to naturally respond, rather than react, to experiences. You will become more insightful and willing to follow your instincts and intuition. Meditation can help you be the person that you want to be, the person you know you can be if only you weren't so stressed out all the time. It doesn't change you or your personality. It just enhances it so you can be the best you possible

5 YOGA

What is yoga? The answer you get depends who you ask. For some, it's a great strength and flexibility workout. For others, it's a way to calm down. For others still, it's a way to re-connect to the greater world around them. Yoga has something for everybody, depending upon what you seek. It's one of the longest surviving holistic health practices in the world, originating about 5,000 years ago in India. It was created to improve health, happiness and connection to higher self.   It was introduced in the US in the late 1800s and is now practiced worldwide by all cultures and religions. The word "Yoga" literally means "to yoke" or "union", referring to connecting the mind, body and spirit. Yoga teaches that when these three things are aligned and working together, life becomes balanced.

There are some misconceptions about yoga that may intimidate those who might otherwise want to give it a try. Here are some facts to help clarify what yoga is and is not:

- Yoga is not a religion. It's a philosophy and lifestyle, open to those of all belief systems and faith.
- One does not have to become a vegetarian or vegan to practice yoga. However, yoga increases awareness of daily choices, including food, that affect health. Eating organic, less or no meat or dairy may become part of your lifestyle as a result.
- You do not need to already be flexible, strong or athletic to do yoga. Anybody can do yoga. It is not about what the pose looks like, but what the pose does for your body, mind and heart that is the key. Though, with regular practice, you will become stronger, more flexible and increase endurance.

The demand for yoga's soothing practices continues to grow, due to ever-increasing amounts of stress and the toll our sedentary, techno-media lifestyle takes on our bodies. Perceived stress activates the sympathetic nervous system. Stress hormones then kick in to increase heart rate, cause shallow breathing, tighten the neck and back muscles, redirect blood from the brain to the arms and legs, and expand eye muscles to heighten peripheral vision. This effect is "fight, flight or freeze" and its purpose is to help you get out of a life-threatening situation. This stress response is great in a true emergency but wasted and even harmful in our day to day lives. As stress hormones keep building up with no natural outlet, we become chronically stressed. This chronic stress is the cause of countless health problems, diseases and disorders.

Yoga, however, short circuits those stress hormones. It activates the parasympathetic nervous system, or "rest and digest" effect. Yoga develops physical and mental focus, strength, balance, flexibility, and overall health. It does more than provide physical and mental benefits, however. Yoga, by connecting the mind to the body, leads you to a natural state of peace and clarity. From this place, you can make decisions that are pro-active responses, rather than knee-jerk reactions to, situations and challenges in your life. Over time, this state of alert calmness will be become your new normal, and this results in greater satisfaction with self, with others, and with life in general.

The sage Patanjali is believed to have written and collected the yoga teachings in a collection called The Yoga Sutras (sutras means thread in Sanskrit), about 2,000 years ago. It was a complete philosophy separated into eight parts, or limbs, to practice for a successful life:

1. Social Restraints (how to treat others)
2. Personal Observances (how to treat oneself)
3. Physical Poses
4. Breathwork
5. Sensory Withdrawal
6. Focused Concentration
7. Effortless Attention
8. Connection to Higher Self

Today, when somebody refers to doing their yoga practice, they are most likely referring to the physical poses, breathwork and/or meditation.

PREPARING FOR PRACTICE

To prepare to do yoga, you need to decide where and what kind of practice you'll be doing. Yoga can be done anywhere, from a chair at the office, to the break room, to your own mat at home. Ideally it will be a place with minimal distractions and some leg and arm room for you to move without bumping into anybody or anything. Wear clothing loose enough that you can move freely, yet not so loose that it hangs off you and gets in your way. Yoga is typically done barefoot, on mats that provide traction to prevent slipping. If you are doing yoga at work, you will obviously need to keep in line with dress code. Yoga props aren't required, but if used they can make poses more comfortable or challenging, depending on your intention and the poses you choose. In addition to yoga mats, common yoga props include foam blocks, cloth straps, bolsters/pillows, and blankets.

YOGA BREATHING TECHNIQUES

The most important yoga prop of all, however, is your breath. This focus and direct cueing of the breath is what makes yoga so different from other workouts and stretching. The breath is considered the anchor that roots the mind into the body, which then makes this work mindful and more effective. It connects the body and mind together in the present moment, activating the relaxation response. The following breathing techniques will help tap into the power of breathing on purpose. They be done as part of a regular yoga practice, or just on their own when you have a few minutes to spare. Choose whichever one seems to meet your needs at that time.

Affirmation Breath

Sit up tall, take a few breaths until you can easily hear your breath. As you inhale, think an affirmation, (i.e., I am strong, I am powerful, etc.), and sense that it is true for you.   As you exhale, let a negative thought (i.e., I can't do this, I'm not good enough, etc.) exit with your exhale, and imagine it losing its power, dissolving into thin air. Continue for 1-5 minutes.

Belly Breath

Sit up tall and take both hands to the belly. Inhale and feel belly filling up with space from the breath. Exhale and feel the belly emptying the space from the breath. Can also be done reclined. Continue 1-5 minutes.

3 Part Breath

- *Sit up tall and take both hands to the belly. Inhale and feel just the belly filling up with space. Exhale and feel the belly emptying the space. Repeat for 3-4 rounds.*
- *Next, place hands at the outside of the ribs. Inhale and feel just the ribs filling up and outward with space. Exhale and feel the ribs emptying the space. Take that through for 3-4 rounds.*
- *Then, place both hands at heart. Inhale and feel just the heart filling up with space. Exhale and feel heart softening. Repeat for 3-4 rounds.*
- *Option: keep one hand at heart, place other hand back at belly. Inhale, feel the belly, then ribs, then heart filling up with space. Exhale, feel heart, then ribs, then belly releasing space. Repeat for 3-4 rounds. Can also be done reclined.*

Cooling Breath

Sit up tall, rest hands palms up on lap. Slightly pucker lips as if drinking through a straw, leaving mouth slightly open. Inhale, feel cool air coming in through the lips. Close the lips and exhale through the nose. Continue for 1–2 minutes.

Make sure that you can always breathe comfortably when doing the poses, and that your body feels good in the poses. If you are forcing or straining yourself, your breath will also become forced and strained-an important clue you are overworking the pose. Don't worry about how 'good' you look in the pose or what others might think. Your health and safety are what is most important.

General Pose Benefits
Certain kinds of poses can have specific physical and energetic effects. For example:

- Standing Poses can help you feel strong, stable and grounded.
- Twists, Core Poses and Heart Openers can give you energy and lift your mood.
- Seated Poses, Forward Folds and Restorative Poses can help you feel calm and reflective.

Pose Length
Unless otherwise indicated, plan to hold each pose in this book for approximately 5-6 rounds of breath, with 1 round being 1 complete inhale and exhale. Make sure your breath keeps flowing when you practice, and that you aren't holding your breath in the poses.

The poses featured in this book can be done in order, as a sequence, or you can pick the ones that work best for you in the moment. Over time you'll naturally start to sense what poses you need as part of your regular practice. Some days you may just choose a few, while other days you may want a longer session. While these poses are intended to help you start to build a regular yoga practice, they aren't a long-term substitute for taking yoga classes at a studio or gym with a teacher who can watch your alignment. If you decide you'd like to explore yoga beyond these pages, I strongly suggest you start working with a teacher.

The Origins of Alignment: Mountain Pose
One pose, Mountain Pose, is considered the primary pose of yoga, with all the other poses following its basic alignment principles. It has a lot of the tenets of 'good posture' that you may have been taught growing up, such as standing tall and keeping a lengthened spine. Both a modified seated version and classic standing version are pictured on the next page.

Mountain Pose

- *Start either seated on chair or standing at front of mat, feet as wide as hip bones and parallel. Knees directly above ankles and pelvis is level (not tipping forwards or back). Hands on thighs, or arms down with palms forward*
- *Inhale, lengthen spine. Ears in line above shoulders.*
- *Exhale, draw navel in. Soften shoulders.*

Seated Mountain

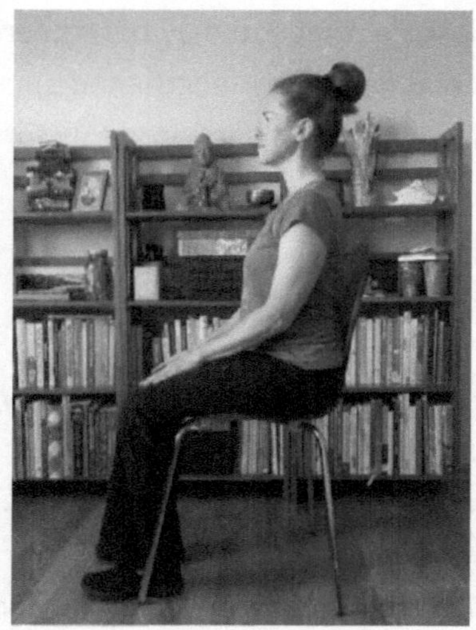

Standing Mountain

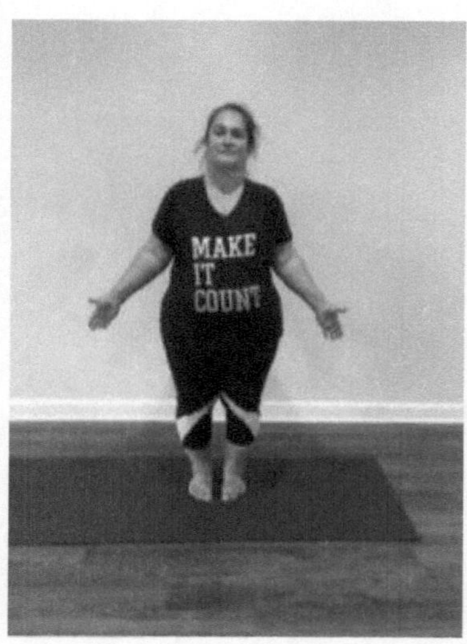

The following poses can be done in the sequence they are shown, or just do which poses you feel serve you best at that time.

Neck Stretch
- *Start either seated on chair, in Easy Pose (pg 9) or Mountain Pose.*
- *Inhale, lengthen spine.*
- *Exhale, softly lower chin toward chest.*

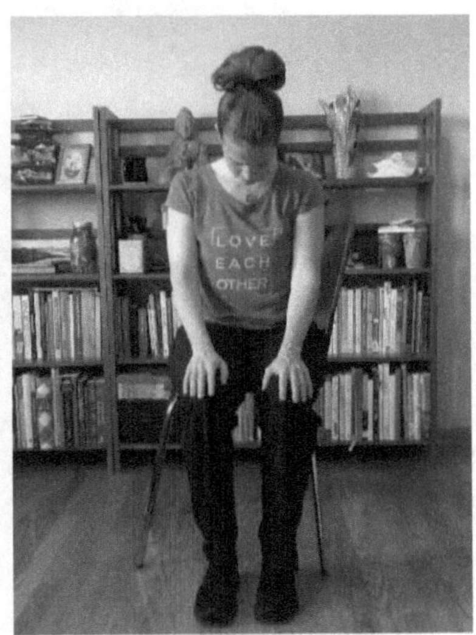

Neck Twist

- *Start either seated on chair, in Easy Pose, or Mountain Pose.*
- *Inhale, lengthen spine.*
- *Exhale, slowly turn head to one side, peek over shoulder (Just head and neck are turned)*

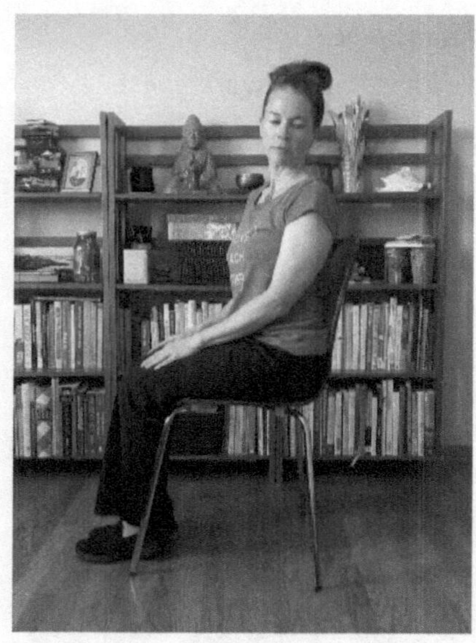

Shoulder Shrugs

- *Start either seated on chair, in Easy Pose, or Mountain Pose.*
- *Inhale, shrug shoulders up toward ears.*
- *Exhale, relax shoulders down to start position.*
- *Repeat shoulder shrug movements 5-6 times.*

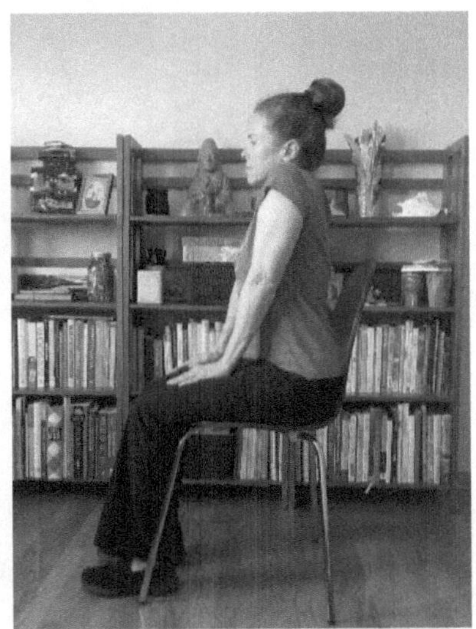

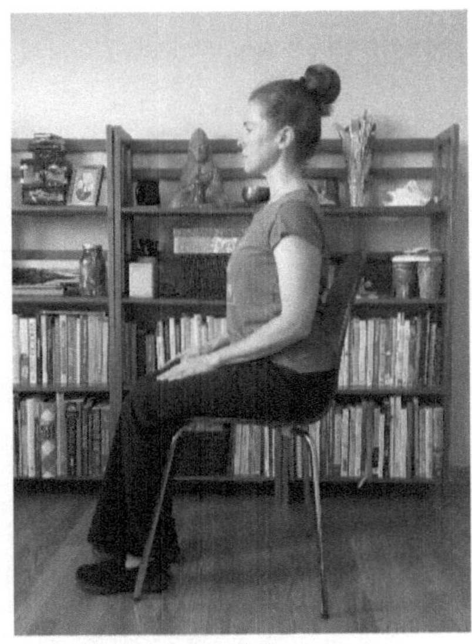

Wrist Warm Up 1

- *Start either seated on chair, in Easy Pose, or Mountain Pose*
- *Inhale, reach one arm forward, fingers up and palm forward.*
- *Exhale, opposite hand slowly presses fingers toward torso.*

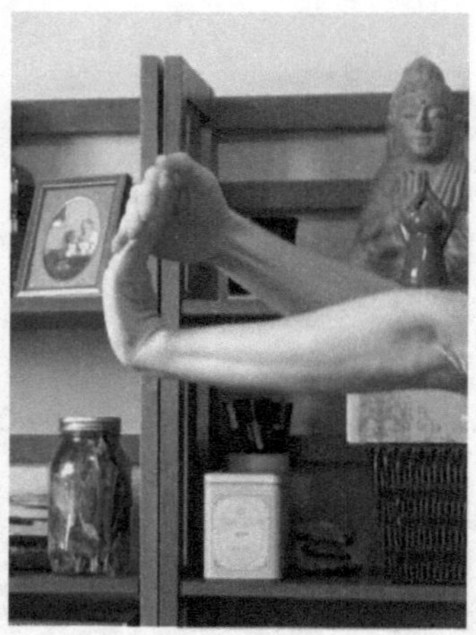

Wrist Warm Up 2

- *Start either seated on chair, in Easy Pose, or Mountain Pose.*
- *Inhale, reach one arm forward, fingers down and palm facing in toward body.*
- *Exhale, opposite hand slowly presses fingers toward torso.*

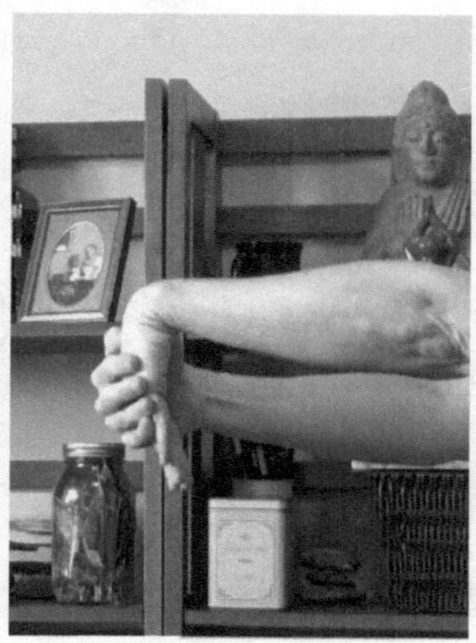

Fingers Warm Up

- *Start either seated on chair, in Easy Pose, or Mountain Pose.*
- *Inhale, raise hand and tap thumb and index finger together a few times.*
- *Exhale, keep tapping the thumb and index finger together.*
- *Repeat the above sequence with thumb and middle finger, then thumb and ring finger, then thumb and pinky finger. Repeat with other hand.*

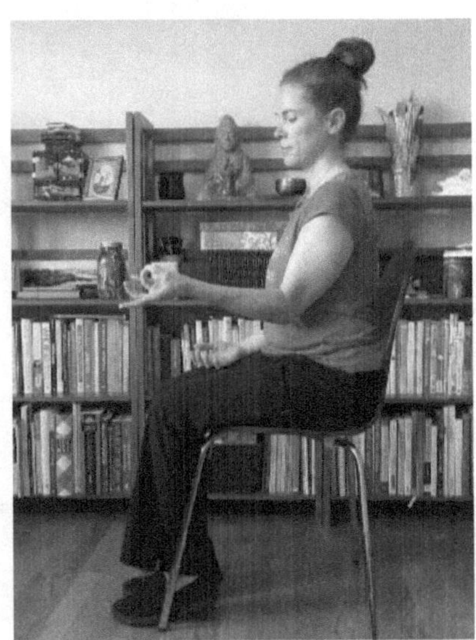

Shoulder Stretch 1 (Heart Opening Clasp)
- *Start either seated on chair, in Easy Pose, or Mountain Pose.*
- *Inhale, lengthen spine and reach arms behind you. Either interlace fingers, press palms into back of chair, or use a strap, belt, towel or computer screen cloth to hold onto (pictured).*
- *Exhale, relax shoulders.*

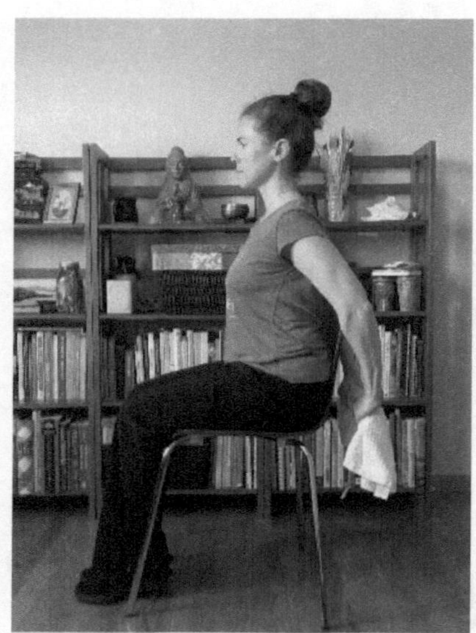

Shoulder Stretch 2 (Cow Face Arms)
- *Start either seated on chair, in Easy Pose, or Mountain Pose. Have a strap, scarf, towel, belt or computer screen cloth in one hand if possible (pictured).*
- *Inhale, lengthen spine and reach hand holding strap upwards.*
- *Exhale, bend elbow and lower strap towards back. Reach other arm behind back to grasp bottom of strap.*
- *Repeat pose to other side.*

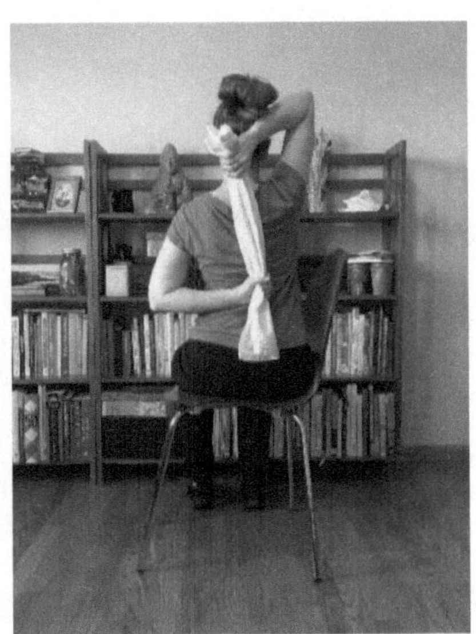

Shoulder Stretch 3 (Eagle Arms)
- *Start either seated on chair, in Easy Pose, or Mountain Pose.*
- *Inhale, lengthen spine, bend elbows. Either cross one elbow on top of the other, or cross opposite forearms.*
- *Exhale, guide hands toward each other. The palms or backs of hands may or may not touch, do not force them.*

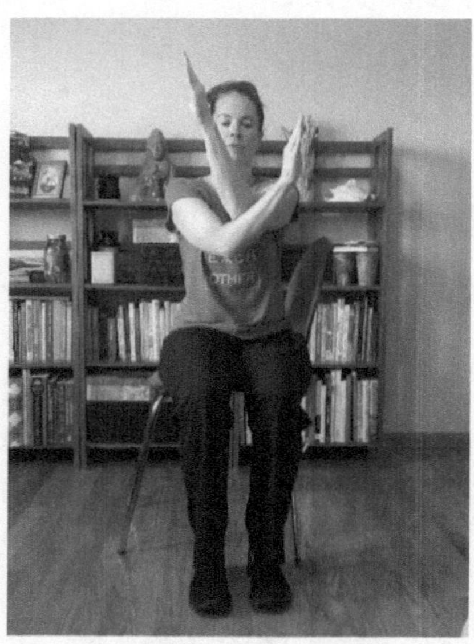

Waist Circles

- *Start either seated on chair, in Easy Pose, or Mountain Pose.*
- *Inhale, lengthen spine, and circle torso forward from right to left, about halfway through one waist circle.*
- *Exhale, circle torso backward from left to right, completing one waist circle.*
- *Repeat waist circles 3-5 times in one direction, then circle 3-5 times in opposite direction.*

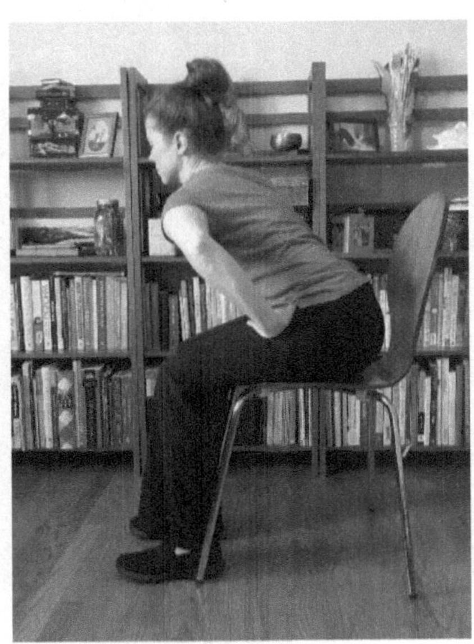

Knee Ups/Single Hip Circles

- *Start seated on chair.*
- *Inhale, lengthen spine, lift foot and bend knee. Take knee in slightly toward torso, then grasp under knee or behind thigh with hands (can use strap, scarf, or towel instead).*
- *Exhale, make 4-6 small hip circles with leg, keep knee facing ceiling.*
- *Repeat with other leg.*

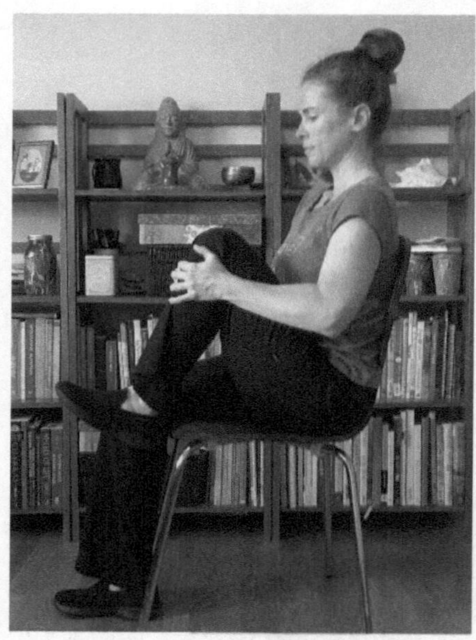

Ankle Stretches

- *Start seated on chair.*
- *Inhale, lengthen spine, lift foot and bend knee. Take knee in slightly toward torso and grasp under knee or behind thigh (can use strap, scarf or towel instead).*
- *Exhale, point toes up toward ceiling, then down toward ground, for 4-6 rounds. Optional ankle circles, 4-6 times per direction.*
- *Repeat with other leg.*

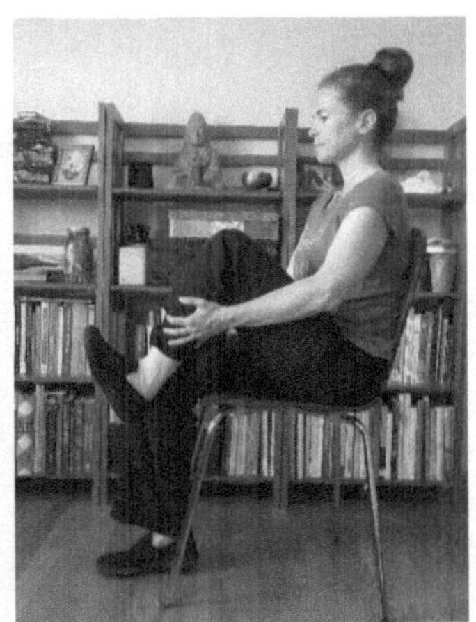

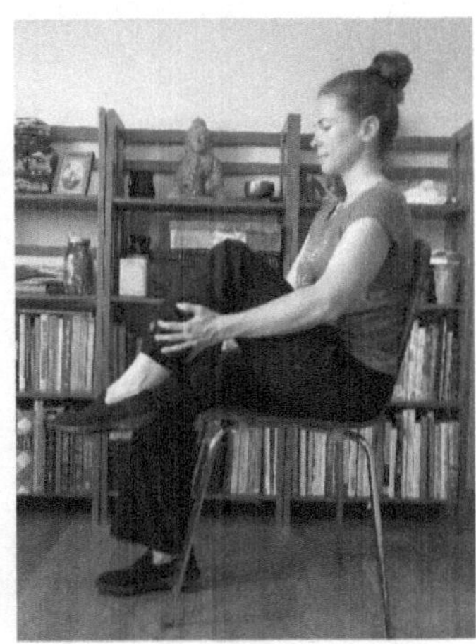

ADDITIONAL YOGA POSES

The following poses have both seated and mat versions pictured.

Cat Pose

- *Start seated or on hands and knees.*
- *Inhale, lengthen spine.*
- *Exhale, round spine, gaze in toward navel.*
- *Repeat 3-5 times, can alternate with cow pose on next page*

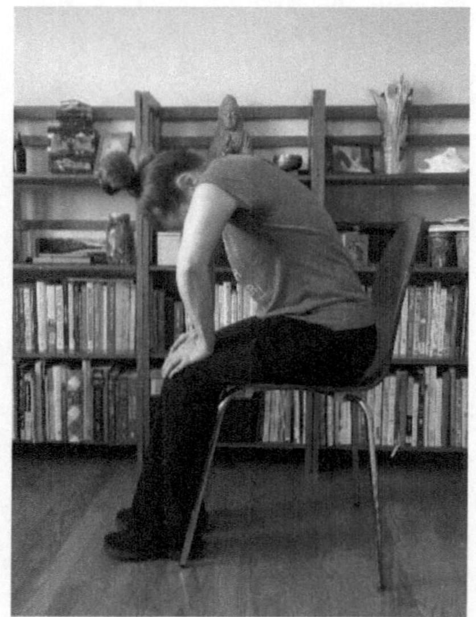

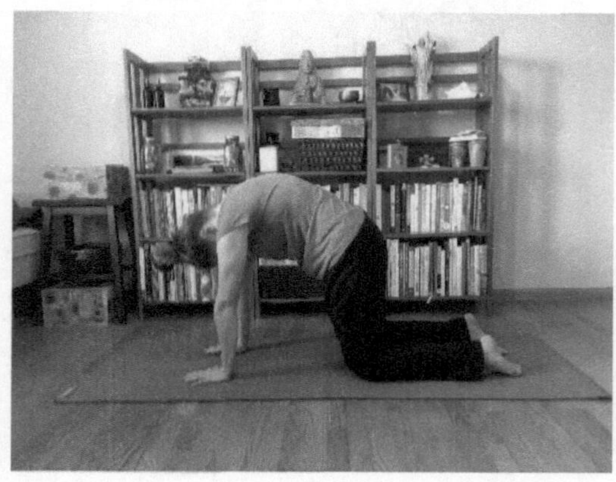

Cow Pose

- *Start seated or on hands and knees.*
- *Inhale, soften belly and comfortably arch spine. Lift tailbone and head.*
- *Exhale, return spine to starting position.*
- *Repeat 3-5 times, can alternate with cat pose on previous page*

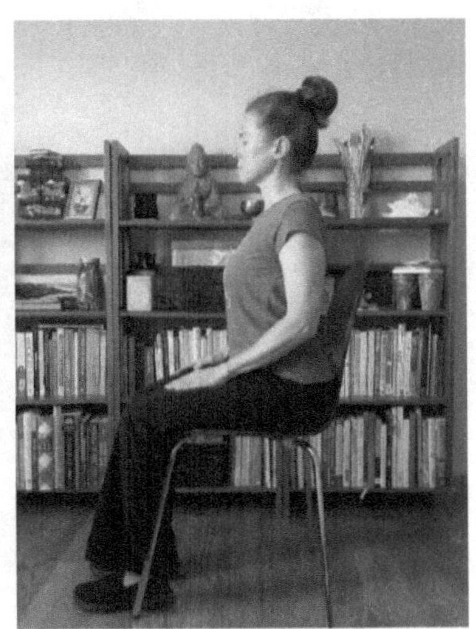

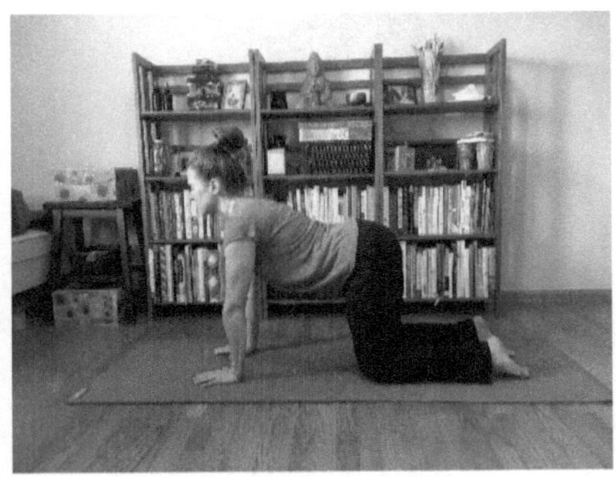

Standing Forward Fold

- *Start in Mountain Pose.*
- *Inhale, lengthen spine. Reach arms up.*
- *Exhale, bend at waist so hands touch the chair back, ground or blocks. Keep spine as long as possible.*

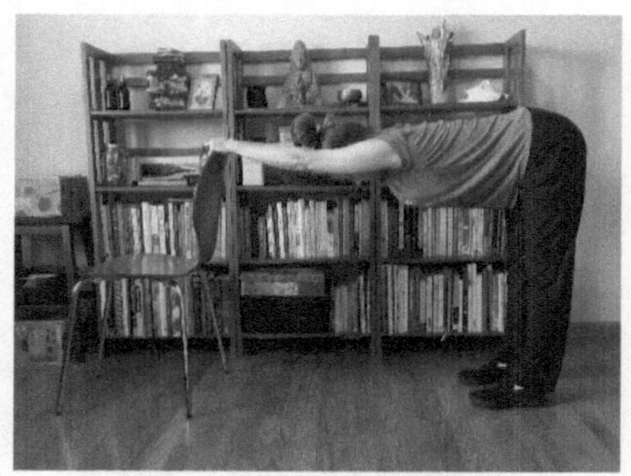

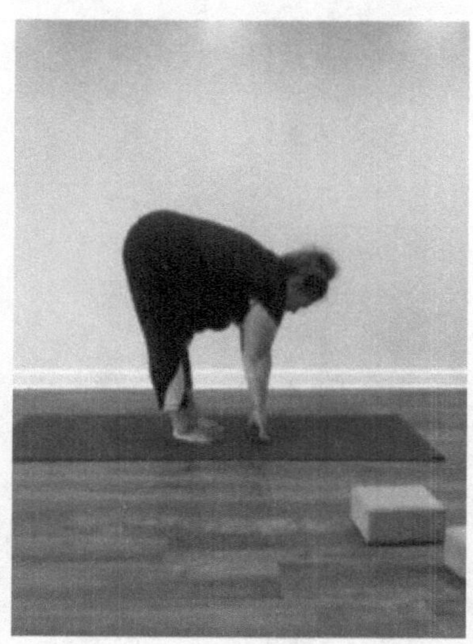

Wide Standing Forward Fold

- *Start in Mountain Pose.*
- *Inhale, lengthen spine, step feet wide apart with toes straight forward. Reach arms up.*
- *Exhale, bend at waist, reach hands down to ground or blocks. Keep spine as long as possible.*

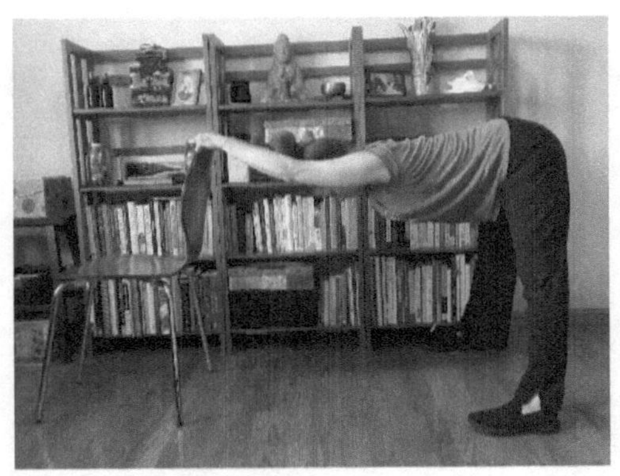

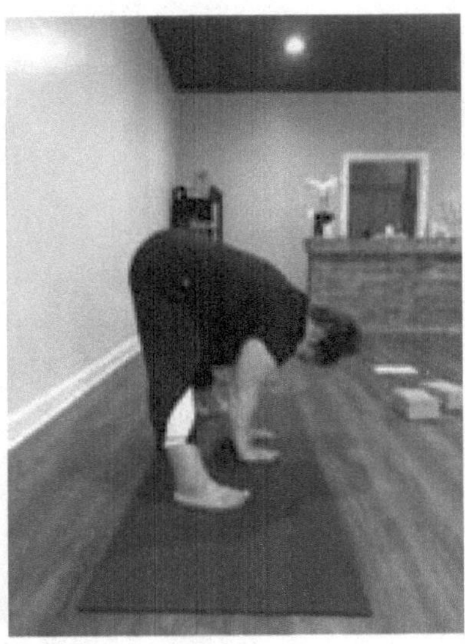

Warrior I

- *Start in Mountain Pose.*
- *Inhale, lengthen spine. Step one foot back. Place hands on chair or desk or reach arms straight up. Press outer edge of back foot down. Back knee faces same direction as back foot.*
- *Exhale, bend front knee, keeping it facing forward and above ankle.*

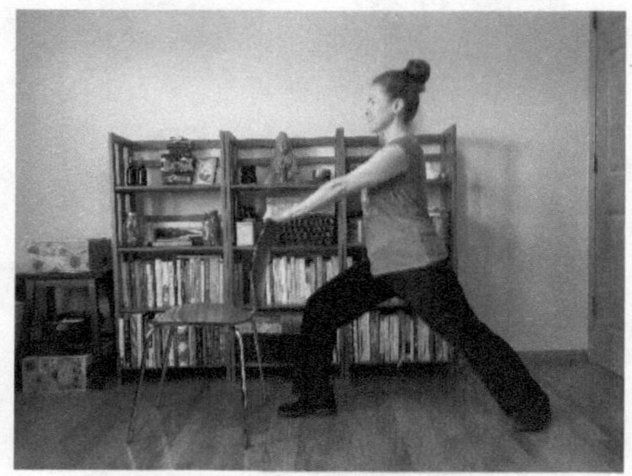

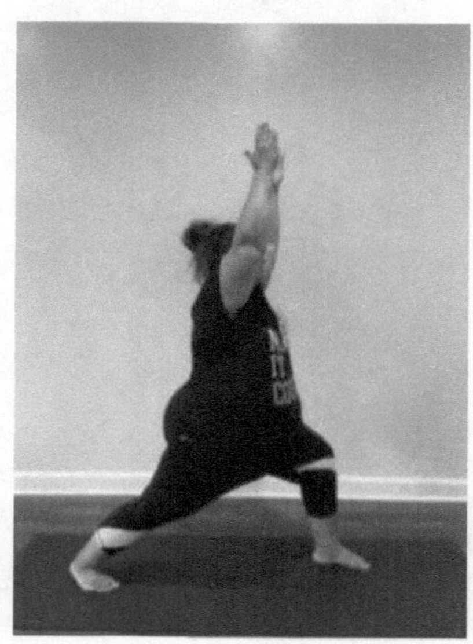

Warrior II

- *Start in Mountain Pose.*
- *Inhale, lengthen spine. Step one foot back, reach that arm back and opposite arm forward to rest on chair or float. Press edge of back foot down. Back knee faces same direction as back foot.*
- *Exhale, bend front knee, keeping it facing forward and above ankle.*

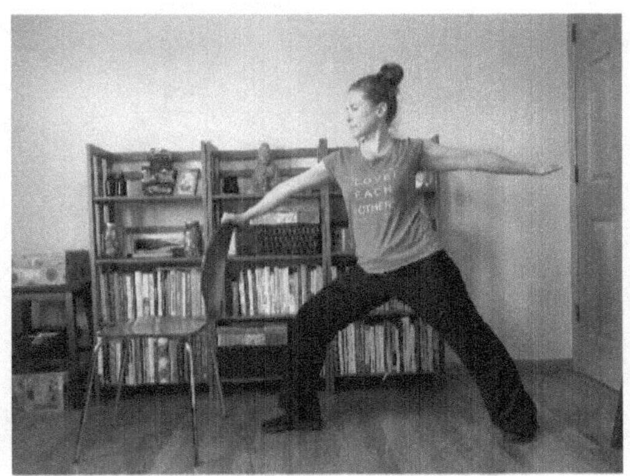

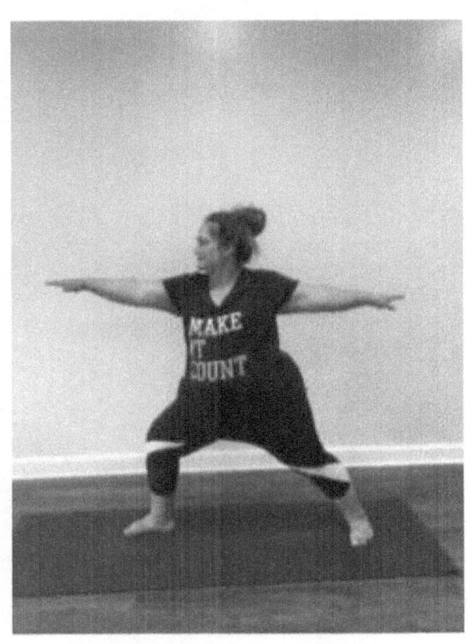

Triangle Pose

- *Start in Warrior II Pose.*
- *Inhale, lengthen spine. Straighten front knee.*
- *Exhale, bend at waist, lower bottom arm down to ground, a block or a chair. Reach opposite hand to hip or straight up. Keep spine as long as possible.*

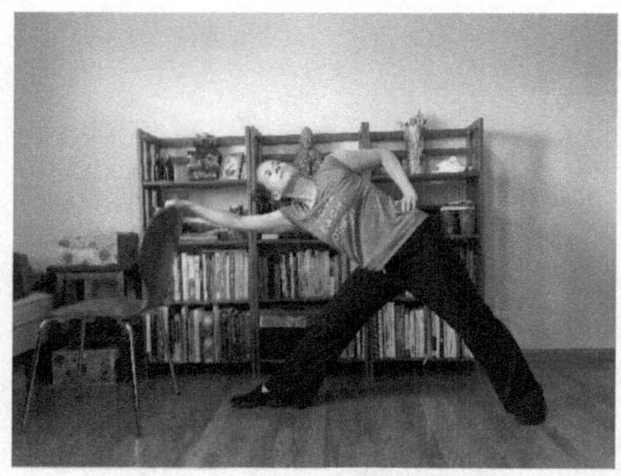

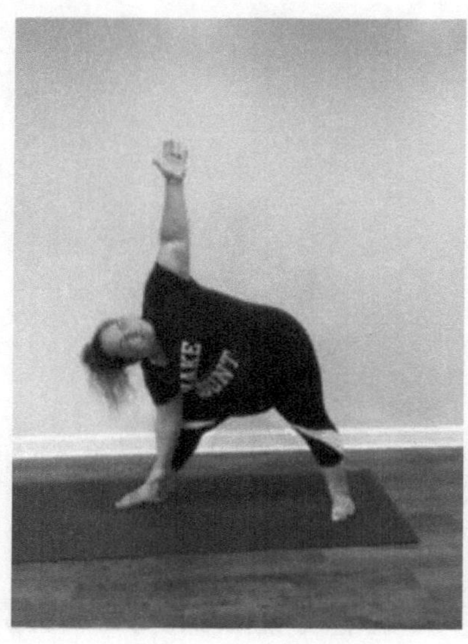

Pyramid Pose

- *Start in Mountain Pose.*
- *Inhale, lengthen spine, step one foot back. Keep torso facing forward and both legs straight. Press outer edge of back foot down. Back knee faces same direction as back foot.*
- *Exhale, bend at waist, reach hands to ground or blocks. Keep spine as long as possible.*

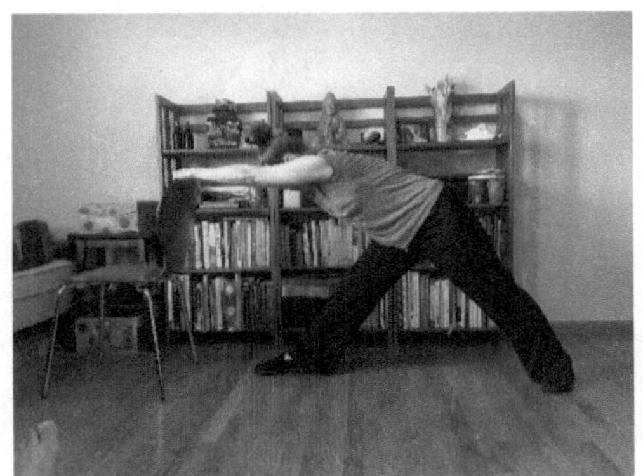

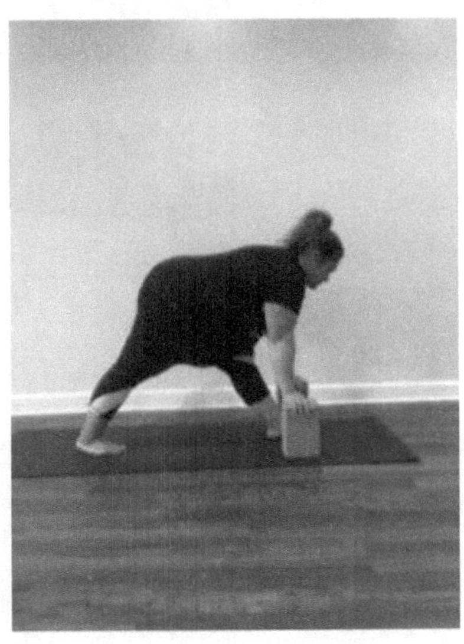

Twist

- *Start seated or in Mountain Pose.*
- *Inhale, lengthen spine.*
- *Exhale, draw navel in and slowly twist torso to left. Hands on chair or palms together at heart. If standing, can slightly bend knees, keeping them facing same direction as toes.*

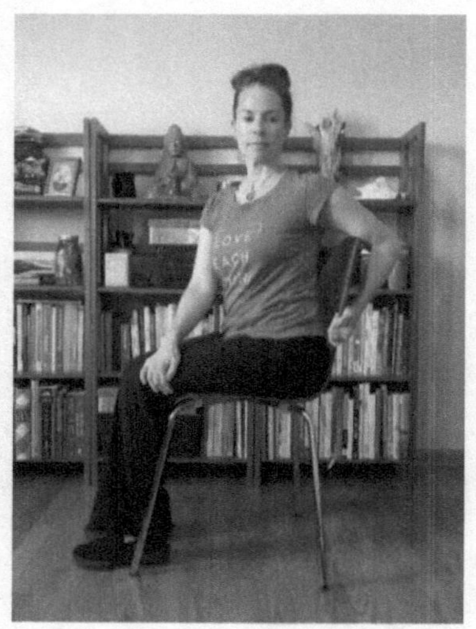

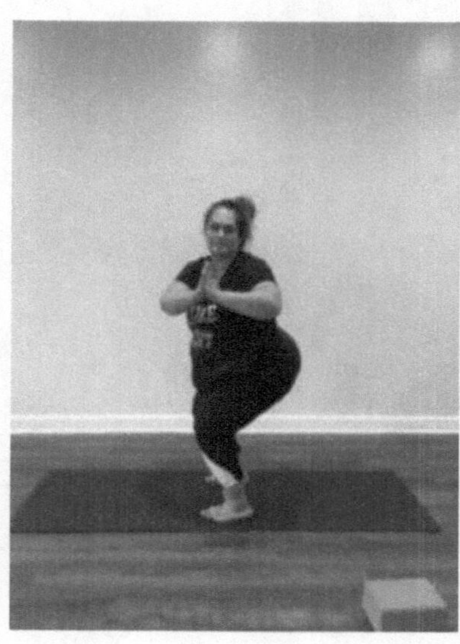

Warrior III

- *Start in Mountain Pose.*
- *Inhale, float one leg straight back off of ground/mat.*
- *Exhale, bend at waist, torso parallel to the ground. Bend elbows and press palms together or reach arms straight forward.*

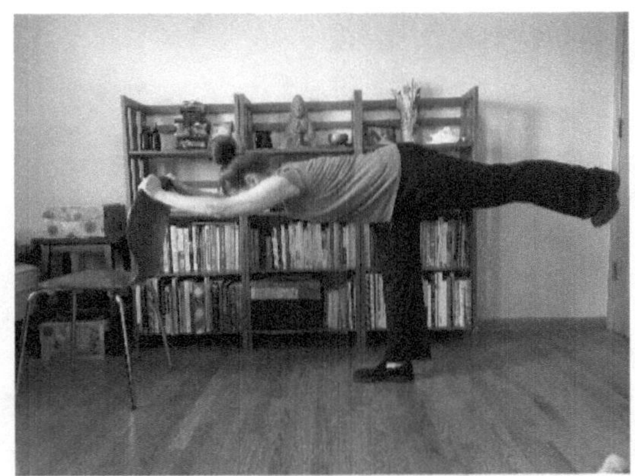

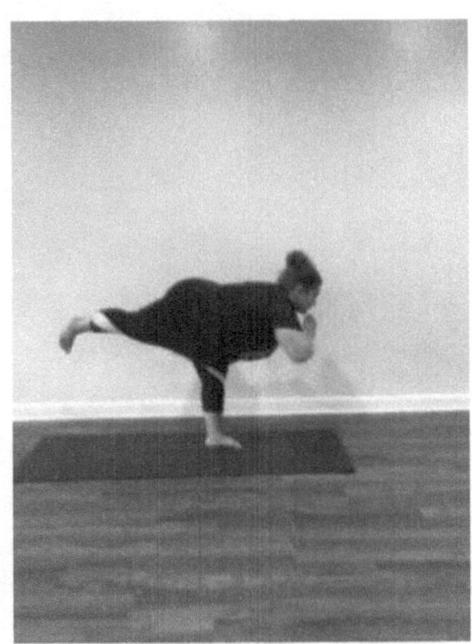

Quad Stretch/Dancer

- *Start in Mountain Pose.*
- *Inhale, lengthen spine.*
- *Exhale, slide one foot back off of ground, bending knee. Grasp foot with same side hand or strap. Reach opposite arm straight forward or rest it on chair. For deeper stretch, bend at waist and press foot higher into hand.*

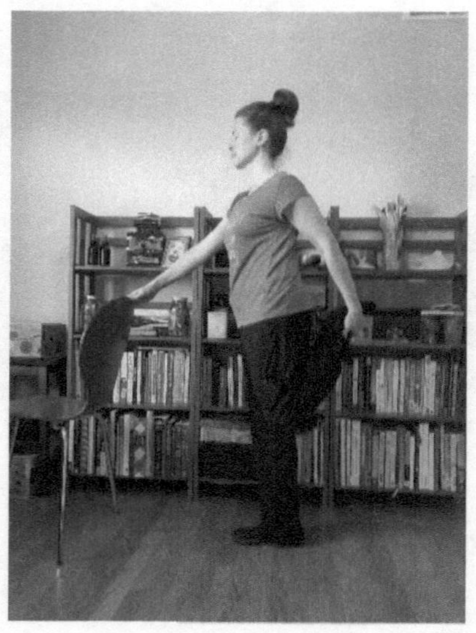

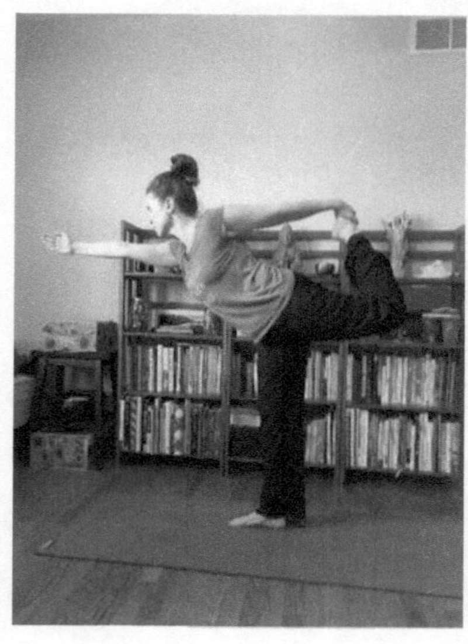

Resting Pose

- *Lie on your back, either with knees bent and resting on chair/bolsters, or knees bent and feet on mat, or legs straight on mat. (Can put bolster under knees if legs straight on mat)*
- *Inhale, feel your spine lengthen.*
- *Exhale, feel your muscles release and relax.*
- *Hold pose for 1-5 minutes.*

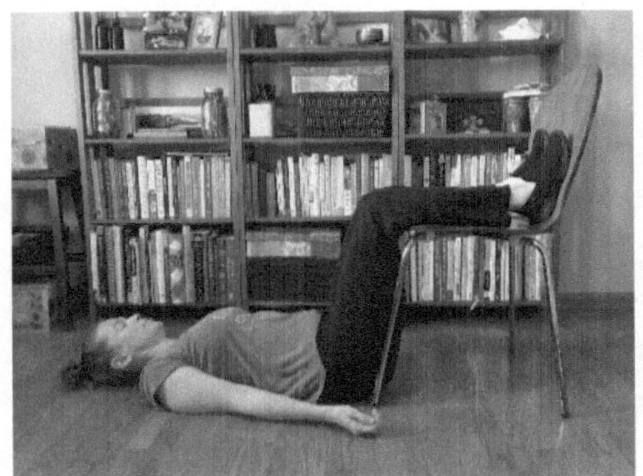

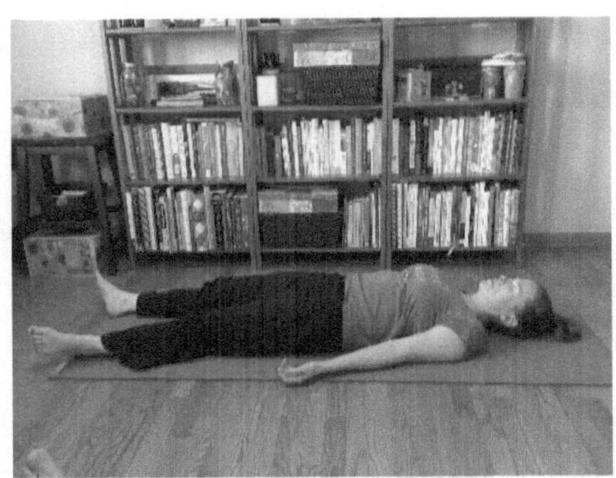

6 AYURVEDA BASICS

Ayurveda is the traditional system of medicine in India. It's also a proactive, mindful and sensory based health care system that can be practiced by anybody, anywhere. Like yoga, Ayurveda looks at a person as multi-layered, considering their body, mind and soul to all be equally important parts. It also recognizes how much we're affected by our environment so bases its interventions on those guidelines. Ayurveda's preventive health practices aim to keep a person's health balanced rather than wait until there is illness or sickness to act.

HISTORY AND ORIGINS

The word Ayurveda is a combination of the Sanskrit *ayur* (life) and *veda* (knowledge), therefore it's knowledge, or science, of life. This blend of philosophy and fact originally developed in India. Now that Westerners are more open to Eastern practices like yoga, Ayurveda is reaching new audiences in the West. They have been called "sister sciences" because they complement one another and were designed to be practiced simultaneously. Ayurvedic studies are now often incorporated into yoga teacher trainings, and several studios offer workshops, classes, and consultation with Ayurvedic specialists. Many people are first introduced to Ayurveda through their yoga teachers or yoga studio. It's now also starting to be regularly featured in magazines, on spa service menus, in blogs, podcasts, and online classes.

THE DOSHAS

Dosha means energy, referring to the different energies both in and around us. Ayurveda recognizes that there are three primary energies, or doshas, that everything in nature has been created from:

- Kapha (Earth and Water)
- Vata (Air and Space)
- Pitta (Fire and Water)

All three of these energies are needed to create and sustain life. The doshas, therefore, can be thought of as operating systems through which all of life's functions and experiences are carried out. Without an amount of each of them present, life could not exist or thrive. These elements also are linked to specific times of day and seasons of the year.

- *Kapha In Nature*: This element expresses itself as solidity, mass and form. It is reflected in nature as planets, mountains, rocks and all solid structures. Internally it is represented in our bones, muscles, tendons, and cartilage. Its qualities are heavy, slow, cold, wet, stable, and dense. Kapha season is winter/early spring. Kapha times of day are 6-10am and 6-10pm.

- *Vata In Nature*: Air is the animating force of life, present in everything that moves. In nature we see this as wind; in the body it is respiration, circulation, and nerve impulses. Its qualities are dry, light, cold, mobile and erratic. Vata season is Fall/Early Winter. Vata times of day are 2-6am and 2-6pm.

- *Pitta In Nature*: Fire is present in everything that generates heat, light, or transformation. We see fire in nature as the sun; inside the body it shows up as digestion, transforming everything going on inside or into the body. Pitta's qualities are light, liquid, hot, sharp, and oily. Pitta Season is Late Spring/Summer. Pitta times of day are 10am-2pm and 10pm-2am.

In addition to the doshas functioning in nature, each of us is born with dominant characteristics in one or more of these areas. Our body type, personality, and other characteristics can be linked back to one or more primary dosha. This mind-body constitution is determined upon conception and is a constant, like a fingerprint. It shows up in physical characteristics, mental and emotional tendencies, and personality traits. Chances are you will recognize one or more of them in yourself or others We each have some of each of these.....the energies of staying steady and strong (kapha), of movement and creativity (vata), and of determination and taking action (pitta). It's just that some of us may be more dominant in one, or sometimes two, of those:

- *Kapha In Us*: Kaphas typically have a strong build, large joints, excellent stamina, round, soft eyes, smooth skin and thick hair. They tend to have good digestion and be heavy sleepers. Kaphas are naturally calm, thoughtful, and loving. They are easygoing, are comfortable with routine, are loyal, patient, steady, and supportive. Too much kapha can result in weight gain, fluid retention, and allergies. They may sleep excessively and/or suffer from asthma, diabetes, and depression. They tend to hold on to things, jobs, and relationships long after they should. They can resist change and be stubborn. They deal with stress by avoiding the situation.

- *Vata In Us*: Vatas usually have a thin, light frame and small joints. They are quick and energetic, though they tire easily. Their skin and hair are light and dry, and their hands and feet are often cold. They are light sleepers with delicate digestion. They love excitement and new experiences. They are creative and energetic, often the life of the party. When a person has too much vata, they may experience unwanted weight loss, constipation, hypertension, arthritis, weakness, restlessness. They are prone to worry and insomnia. They quickly become anxious when experiencing stress.

- *Pitta in Us:* Pittas are usually medium size and weight, sometimes with reddish thinning hair. They tend to be naturally warm, have excellent digestion, and sleep well. When in balance, pittas have a glowing complexion, lots of energy, strong appetite, sharp wit and focus. They are good decision makers, teachers, and speakers. Excess pitta can mean skin rashes, burning sensations, peptic ulcers, digestive problems and excessive heat. They can get short-tempered and argumentative. When stressed, they become quickly irritated or angry.

Curious if you're kapha, vata or pitta dominant? There are several free online quizzes you can take created by various Ayurvedic doctors, practitioners and companies. Simply search 'free dosha quiz'.

CLUES TO DOSHA IMBALANCE

When there is too much of one dosha, we call that dosha imbalanced, or out of balance. When there is an imbalance (too much) of one dosha, a person builds up stagnant physical and/or energetic residue called ama. This results in dis-ease (discomfort) that, if not dealt with, could eventually result in disease. Regardless of one's individual dosha, general triggers to excess amounts of a dosha include changes between seasons, lifestyle choices, relationships, career or schooling, food...really, just about anything a person experiences through their senses during the day. On the other hand, when all three of these elements work together and remain in the best balance for that person, they support one another, sustaining the individual with radiant health.

As a general guideline, we rebalance the imbalanced dosha by bringing in its opposite qualities. A lot of Ayurvedic interventions are things that you probably already knew, and it was just time to be reminded again. There's a reason why this has stood the test of time....it just makes sense.

Please note: Since Ayurveda is a comprehensive health system, it can be used in many contexts. Its use ranges from tips and tools that can be used by the layperson as self-care to maintain their own health and wellness, all the way to working with an medically trained and licensed

Ayurvedic practitioner who performs specific diagnostic tests (i.e., pulse reading) and prescribes courses of treatment or remedies such as herbs. The information presented in this book is being shared in the first context. If you decide you'd like to learn more about Ayurveda, or even possibly work with a trained practitioner, I'll provide books, websites, and a national listing of qualified Ayurvedic practitioners through NAMA in the Resources section

TOO MUCH KAPHA: CLUES

Body: Feeling of heaviness; slow metabolism; weight gain; weakness; sweet tooth; indigestion; asthma; colds or flu; coughs; runny nose; congestion; sinus problems; cold sweats.

Mind: Sluggish; brain fog; unmotivated; oversleeping; excessive fatigue; laziness; depression; envious; clingy; complacent; possessive.

Behaviors/Environment: Eating heavy foods like ice cream; overeating; emotional eating; stagnant lifestyle; repressing emotions.

What Can Help: Eat in a loving environment; avoid excessive periods of time sitting, journal to release emotions; wake up early; go to bed early; avoid excessive naps; dress or decorate with bright colors like red, orange, yellow and purple; choose cardio exercise like running or hiking; listen to rhythmic, lively music; change up your daily routine; avoid heavy, cold desserts; eat light, warm, foods such as soups and cooked vegetables.

TOO MUCH VATA: CLUES

Body: Difficulty making or keeping eye contact; excessive movement/can't stay still; constipation; gas and bloating; chronic fatigue; low energy; intolerance of cold; excessive thirst; irregular appetite; unintentional weight loss; dry skin; insomnia; no appetite.
Mind: Anxious; nervous; afraid to be alone; insecure; restless;

hyperactive; grandiose thinking; impulsive; disorganized; indecisive; talking fast; impatient; giddiness; racing thoughts; unwilling or able to keep commitments; forgetfulness.

Behaviors/Environment: Times of transitions (i.e., starting or ending school, relationships, birth or death, moving, seasons, big events); eating a lot of dry foods like cereal, raw vegetables and crackers; cold food or drinks; going to sleep after 10:30pm; excessive physical activity; excessive noise; lack of creative opportunities.

What Can Help: Eat warm, grounding food like soups and stews; bedtime 10:30pm or earlier; regular sleep and meal schedule (including weekends); completing tasks; dress or decorate with relaxing earth tones, pastels, browns and warm yellows; spend time in nature, listen to calming music or nature sounds; take naps; stay warm; use scents like lavender and cinnamon; choose confidence and strength building exercise like martial arts, yoga or self-defense workouts.

TOO MUCH PITTA: CLUES

Body: Intense hunger; excessive thirst; hyperacidity; ulcers; inflammation; sensitivity to spicy foods; skin rashes; hemorrhoids; body odor; excessive sweating; sensitivity to light; strong appetite; becomes irritable when hungry.

Mind: Overly competitive; perfectionistic; impatient; judgmental; irritability/anger; aggressive; manipulative; jealous.

Behavior/Environment: Excess hunger; spicy foods; eating while angry or upset; too much caffeine; over working; too much heat; loud and aggressive environments.

What Can Help: Eat in a peaceful environment; keep snacks handy to avoid excessive hunger; avoid hot, spicy foods; eat cooling foods like sweet fruits, salads, and cooked vegetables; choose cool colors like blue, green and white; listen to calming string instrumental music; laugh, smile and have fun; take cooler showers; spend time walking in the moonlight; avoid competitive sports; avoid getting overheated; reduce time in the sun during peak hours (10am-2pm), choose cooler exercise like swimming or running during cooler parts of the day.

7 AYURVEDIC MEAL PLANNING

One only needs to look to nature to see its life force, or prana, shining bright. It makes sense that the closer we are to nature in our food choices, the more we keep that inherent state of health and vitality. We truly are and become what we eat. It's also important that we're in the right frame of mind when we eat, otherwise we can't properly digest our food and the healthy choices you made when meal planning will be for naught. To lower toxins and help your metabolism work at its best, it may be time to reconsider what, when and how you eat.

FOOD AND THE DOSHAS

Ayurveda considers food more than a source of energy and nourishment. It looks at a food's flavor profile and its ability to create heat, cold, dryness or moisture in the body. If we have too much of something going on, it suggests foods with the opposite qualities to rebalance us. This is why warm stew is calming when there's too much anxious (cold and dry) vata, why ice cream on a summer day cools aggravated (hot and damp) pitta, and why a light stir fried veggie meal lightens lethargic (cold and damp) kapha. So how can you use this for some quick meal planning? Just keep the following suggestions in mind and remember the formula: choose foods with the opposite qualities to balance out when you're feeling too much of something (think of it like a teeter-totter). Notice the effects when you follow these guidelines. You'll start to figure out which of these foods works best for you and when.

Feeling anxious or distracted? You might have too much vata going on. More sweet, sour or salty foods may help.

Feeling irritable or agitated? You might have too much pitta going on. More sweet, bitter or astringent foods may help.

Feeling sluggish or lethargic? You might have too much kapha going on.

More of pungent, salty or astringent foods may help.

- *Sweet foods* can help rebuild tissues and promote longevity. Examples of sweet foods include wheat, rice, dairy, cereals, dates, pumpkins, maple syrup, and licorice root.
- *Sour foods* can increase appetite and improve digestion. Examples of sour foods include lemon, vinegars, pickled and fermented foods, tamarind, and wine.
- *Salty foods* can help with electrolyte balance and nutrient absorption. Examples of salty foods include sea vegetables, sea salt, tamari, black olives, Himalayan salt, and rock salt
- *Pungent* foods are clearing and stimulating. Examples of pungent foods include hot peppers, ginger, onions, garlic, mustard, and hot spices.
- *Bitter foods* are detoxifying. Examples of bitter foods include raw green vegetables, turmeric, and green, black and most herbal teas.
- *Astringent* foods purify and strengthen. Examples of astringent foods include unripe bananas, green grapes, pomegranates, cranberries, green beans, alfalfa sprouts, and okra.

Your food will have more nutritional bang for its buck when it meets the following guidelines:

- Eat unprocessed, organic, whole foods whenever you can.
- Eat homemade foods whenever you can, so you know what's actually in it.
- Lightly cooked foods are preferable to raw or overcooked foods since they're easier to digest.
- Drink less ice-cold beverages because they interfere with digestion.
- Choose foods from all colors of the rainbow to make sure you get the range of vitamins, minerals, nutrients and phytochemicals that are provided by each color group.

ADDITIONAL MINDFUL EATING TIPS FOR WORK AND HOME:

- Don't eat when upset-stress interferes with digestion. If you have complaining co-workers on break with you that get you riled up, change the topic, put on ear buds, or eat somewhere else if possible (your car, etc). If you're not sure how true this is, notice the differences you feel afterwards when eating in a calm environment; eating with someone who is complaining; eating when you are the one complaining.
- Eat at a leisurely pace, using the senses to notice all aspects of your food.
- Bring meals to work so you don't have to rush out to grab something, then rush to finish it before your break ends.
- Don't overeat; leave a bit of room in your stomach to help digest the meal.
- Sit quietly for a minute or two after finishing your meal.
- Make sure you actually bring food you actually like to work, so you're not tempted to run out to fast food restaurants on your break, or look at your co-workers' food with meal-envy and end up stopping for french fries on the way home (yes, I've done this.)
- If you know there's a regular treat day (ie, Donut Friday, Bagel Monday) and are trying to lower/cut these foods out, bring a reasonable portion of something you actually like BETTER instead, so you don't feel tempted by the treat. Even if it's a homemade brownie, chances are since it's homemade it will be better for you, and the smaller portion will stave off mindlessly grabbing the donuts as they sit there during your shift (yes, I've done this too)
- If you decide to indulge in the above mentioned treat, truly savor it by taking your time and enjoying every bite. Do NOT waste time with guilt or regret. If you choose to have it, then completely choose it and commit to that choice. Life is too short for anything less.

8 SCHEDULE: THE AYURVEDIC CLOCK

Ever wonder why you get that 3pm slump, that second wind after 10pm or wake up unexpectedly at 2am? It's likely that you're out of rhythm with the Ayurvedic clock. A primary way that Ayurveda aligns us with nature is by recognizing that each section of the day has a specific type of dosha that dominates it. This is determined by the sun's placement during that time of day. One part of the day is supposed to be slower, another part more focused, and a third part more creative. Once we know this, we can use this to our best advantage-to be more productive at work, as well as happier and healthier throughout the day.

Our brains take their cues from the sun's position as well and signal our bodies to perform various functions based on time of day and the light of the sun. You might have already learned this somewhere along the way how these circadian rhythms do their best to keep us on schedule with all aspects of functioning. Modern life hasn't really accounted for these old natural rhythms, though. We have gotten away from them and instead developed new, though not necessarily better, habits based on how society functions now. These routines, unfortunately, just end up working against us, contributing to stress, exhaustion, and eventual disease. To restore our health, then we simply take our cues from the sun. These scheduling tricks are basically aces up your sleeve. A better use of your time, of when to do things. When to rest, when to play, when to work, when to sleep.... really, a better way to live. Not coincidentally, this also follows what is considered the successful formula for life balance: allowing at least some time for all the above. Here's the daily dosha breakdown:

Kapha Shifts-Early morning and early evenings, 6-10am and 6-10pm, are kapha times. This is when the sun comes up, signaling the body it's time to rise. This is a slow moving, gentle time where we gradually increase the intensity of our thoughts and actions. Important self-care practices that help us with this include meditation, exercise, and eating a light breakfast before starting work or tackling other planned activities. This provides energy that you'll draw upon as your day continues. Tasks completed during this time should be simple, routine assignments or projects that continue to gently wake up the brain. The biggest challenges of this time can either be waking up exhausted or skipping your self-care and jumping right into your to do list, which just leaves you depleted later. At night, this time functions in reverse. Meals and activities during this time should therefore also be light, to gradually wind you down, relax your body and mind, and prepare for sleep.

Pitta Shifts -Later morning/early afternoon and later evening, 10am-2pm and 10pm-2am, are pitta times. You might have already noticed that 10am is when many people naturally become more productive. You've checked emails and get that morning second wind to tackle bigger projects. This is when the sun shines brightest, so our drive, motivation and energy tend to be strongest. This is the time of day you want to schedule tasks to be completed. 12pm is when we're supposed to eat our biggest meal, smack dab in the middle of that productive pitta time. It's very easy to ignore this, especially if you're in a zone or on a deadline and think it's no big deal to skip lunch if you have a bigger dinner. What this does, however, is make you crabby, lowers your concentration, and leaves you with undigested food in your stomach before bed, interfering both with sleep and proper digestion. So, make time for it, even if it's just stepping away from a meeting or conference call for 10 minutes. (You'll be more productive and pleasant to be around). At night, pitta time is when we get the most useful sleep. Though we think of sleep as a restful, relaxing time, the truth is that the body and mind are getting a lot done in this state. Falling asleep between 10-10:30pm is the commonly agreed upon timeframe to ensure you get the most benefits from this phase.

Vata Shifts- Late afternoon and very early morning, from 2-6pm and 2am-6pm, are vata times. It's the time of movement, of energy, of creativity. Many people get the 2pm crash or slump, even more so if they didn't eat lunch or are trying to stay alert with coffee or energy drinks. For all of us, though, there tends to be a natural energetic shift that happens at 2pm. (Seriously, today or tomorrow, see if you can notice it). This is a great time to transition with a cup of tea or going for a quick walk…. something that allows you a couple of minutes to check in with yourself and acknowledge that you are shifting to a different part of your day. This time works well as more of a creative space in your schedule, a good time for brainstorming and idea sessions. If possible, leave work at a decent hour (by 5 or 6pm) and have a lighter dinner so it's completely digested by the time you go to sleep. Regarding vata's second shift, this 2am time tends to be the time when people wake for no apparent reason. Having prepared accordingly by winding down your evening and gotten to sleep before the pitta window closed helps minimize this 2am wake up call.

HEALTHY SLEEP

A key component of any successful retreat is plenty of time for rest, relaxation, and more rest! Restful sleep is essential for health and longevity. The hours between 10pm and 2am are the most important hours for sleep, as this is when the body and mind digest the day and make necessary repairs.

Do your best to be in bed with the lights out by 10:30pm to get the best rest possible. This can take awhile to wrap your head around if you're one of the many people who routinely stay up past midnight. I'm one of those former night owls, and I acknowledge it can take awhile to get into this habit. But it's absolutely worth it. You'll feel better during your day, and have more energy, focus and productivity in your work. If you are try and find difficulty staying with this, make the shift more subtle-move all parts of your bedtime routine earlier by just half an hour per week, until you are in bed by 10:30pm (or earlier if you like). In addition to regulating the bedtime schedule, these tips can help establish a routine that helps you fall-and stay-asleep:

- Take a hot bath an hour before bed, using essential oil like lavender, sandalwood or vanilla.

- After your bath, have a cup of hot tea or warm milk.
- If your mind is very active, journal for a few minutes before bed. This downloads those perseverative or repeating thoughts, so you don't keep replaying them when you shut your eyes.
- Make a brief short to-do list for the next day, to prevent those nagging thoughts that might keep you up ("I have to remember to…."). Knowing they're on the list takes them off your brain for the time being. DO NOT START ACTUALLY DOING THE LIST OR THINKING ABOUT THE ITEMS ON THE LIST. If this step ends up being distracting, another option is to make the to-do list at your work station before you leave it for the day so that it's waiting for you.
- Read a few minutes' worth of inspirational or spiritual literature. Books with short chapters, or magazines with brief articles work well. Make sure this is an actual paper book, however, not a kindle or iPad, as the light can disrupt natural rhythms. (see next two suggestions)
- Keep the screens off once you're in bed-don't watch television, work, or otherwise use your computer or phone while you are in bed. This keeps you focused on the outside world and not on preparing yourself to rest.
- Turn off electronics at least one hour before bedtime, to give yourself time to unplug and retreat and lower the effects of their blue light, which can interfere with sleep.
- Once in bed, close your eyes and simply feel your body. Start from the crown of the head and go all the way to the tips of the toes, scanning for any areas of tightness that you can breathe softness into. If you notice tension in specific parts of the body, briefly contract (tighten) the muscles, then relax them.
- If you have trouble falling asleep, listen to a guided visualization, just noticing the natural ebb and flow of your breath until you fall asleep.

9 CALM, COOL AND CHEERFUL: AYURVEDIC MOOD STRATEGIES

Ayurveda teaches us that we are nature, so it makes sense we to use nature's lessons and simple rhythms to stay healthy, especially when it comes to maintaining mood balance. We connect to the world around us through sight, sound, smell, taste, touch, and non-verbal communication. Ayurveda activates these senses through deliberate choices and intentional connections. The following guidelines can be applied to yourself or others.

Possible Kapha Imbalance/Too Much Earth: If someone is always experiencing nausea, breathing difficulties or needs to sleep a lot, they may be suffering from a kapha imbalance. It also can show up as lethargy, excessive mucus discharge and circulation problems.

To Cheer Kapha:

- *Colors:* vibrant and bright, i.e. orange, red, yellow
- *Music*: invigorating lively
- *Tastes/spices*: have heat, i.e., chilis, garlic, onion
- *Scents:* cinnamon, ginger, juniper, clary sage
- *Interactions:* Somebody with too much kapha responds well to lively, energetic words and actions

Possible Vata Imbalance/Too Much Wind: A person who is very thin, has rough flaky skin, is anxious and worried, could possibly have a vata imbalance.

To Calm Vata:

- *Colors:* earthy and pastel, i.e. khaki, grey, olive, light pinks, yellows and greens
- *Music:* calming and relaxing, classical music, slower paced

- *Tastes*: spices: grounding and earthy, i.e., cumin, cardamom, cinnamon
- *Scents*: geranium, lavender, vanilla
- *Interactions:* Somebody with too much vata responds well to nurturing, soothing words and actions.

Possible Pitta Imbalance/Too Much Fire: An imbalance in pitta might be indicated by someone who seems to be angry all the time, or impatient and frustrated. Physically they may suffer from rashes or other types of skin eruptions. They may also have digestive problems, including heartburn or even ulcers.

To Cool Pitta:

- *Colors:* cool and calm, i.e. blues and greens
- *Music:* soft, ethereal, nature sounds, wind chimes, flute, water
- *Tastes/spices* are cooling and soothing, i.e. fennel, coriander, cilantro
- *Scents:* jasmine, neroli, patchouli, mandarin.
- *Interactions:* Somebody with too much pitta responds well to specific, direct words and actions that leave little ambiguity or question about expectations

10 YOUR TURN: CHOOSE YOUR SELF-CARE STAPLES

The self-care practices of meditation, yoga and Ayurveda build on each other. Study and practice of one of these enhances study and practice of the others.   Choose whichever of these works best for you, whether it's just one tip or trick, or several daily rituals……whatever best fits in to your life and what you need.

Take a few minutes now to imagine a typical day. As you imagine this day, set an intention for honoring yourself, and taking time to nurture yourself, whatever form that ends up taking. Spend a few minutes on each segment of your day, from waking, to breakfast, to commute (if you have one), to work, lunch and break time, to back home again, to dinner, to winding down the day and preparing for sleep. If your day goes in a slightly different order from what I just outlined, imagine that instead. Look for possible pockets where some of these strategies naturally fit in. For any that you might feel a lot of resistance to, don't focus on those right now.   Keep attention instead on what feels like a good fit. Eventually, those techniques that seemed a bit daunting or foreign may pique your curiosity, and you may give those a try. No need to overwhelm, there's plenty of time for you to design your ideal self-care routine. What matters is your willingness to try, your understanding that you ARE worth this time, and that when you take care of yourself EVERYBODY benefits. You become that version of yourself that was always there, that best version that you always knew you could be.

Yoga classes typically end with the greeting Namaste, which translates as 'the unique light that shines in me honors the unique light that shines in you'. So thank you once more, for sharing this journey with me, and for making your self-care a priority. Namaste.

REFERENCES & RESOURCES

BOOKS

Chopra, Deepak, MD. *Perfect Health*. New York, NY: Three Rivers Press; 1991, R 2000.

Chopra, Deepak, MD & Simon, David. *The Seven Spiritual Laws of Yoga*. Hoboken, NJ: John Wiley and Sons, Inc; 2004.

Davidji. *Secrets of Meditation*. Carlsbad, CA: Hay House Inc; 2012

Desikachar, TKV. *The Heart of Yoga: Developing A Personal Practice*. Rochester, VT: Inner Traditions International; 1995.

Dispenza, Joe, DC. *Becoming Supernatural: How Common People Are Doing The Uncommon*. Carlsbad, CA: Hay House Publishing; 2019.

Kabat-Zinn Jon, University of Massachusetts Medical C. *Full Catastrophe Living: Using the Wisdom of Your Body and Mind to Face Stress, Pain, and Illness*. New York, N.Y.: Delta Trade Paperbacks; 2005.

Kshirsagar, Suhas, MD. *The Hot Belly* Diet. New York, NY: Atria Books; 2014

Lad, Vasant, MD. *Ayurveda: The Science of Self-Healing*. Santa Fe, NM: Lotus Press; 1984.

Rosenthal, Joshua. *Integrative Nutrition*. New York, NY: Integrative Nutrition Publishing; 2017

Satchinanada, Sri Swami. *The Yoga Sutras of Patanjali*. Ashland, OH: Integral Yoga Publications; 2012

Silcox, Katie. *Healthy Happy Sexy: Ayurveda Wisdom for Modern Women*. Hillsboro, OR: Beyond Words; 2015.

Yarema, Thomas MD et al. *Eat Taste Heal: An Ayurvedic Guidebook and Cookbook for Modern Living.* Kapaa, HI: Five Elements Press; 2010

ARTICLES

8 Steps to Establish a Daily Meditation Practice. (2016, October 11).(n.d.) Retrieved July 25, 2019, from http://www.chopra.com/articles/8-steps-to-establish-a-daily-meditation-practice#sm.000011af3bkgbdfkaw6j53wcpiqs6

New Study Shows Correlation Between Employee Engagement And The Long Lost Lunch Break (2018, May 29) (n.d.). Retrieved July 25, 2019 from https://www.forbes.com/sites/alankohll/2018/05/29/new-study-shows-correlation-between-employee-engagement-and-the-long-lost-lunch-break/amp/

Putting Ayurvedic Theory Into Practice. (2014, March 18). Retrieved July 25, 2019, from http://www.integrativehealthcare.org/mt/archives/2011/03/putting_ayurved.html

Reduced rates of death, heart attack and stroke. (n.d.). Retrieved July 25, 2019, from http://www.tm.org/american-heart-association

Want more productive employees? Encourage Self Care (2017), February 14th. (n.d.). Retrieved July 25, 2019, from https://www.huffpost.com/entry/want-more-productive-employees-encourage-self-care_b_58a3763be4b0e172783aa19e

WEBSITES

http://www.ayurvedanama.org (National Avurvedic Medical Association), includes listings of Ayurvedic Practitioners

http://chopra.com (Chopra Center)

http://www.mapi.com (Maharishi Ayurvedia Products International)

https://www.yogajournal.com (Yoga Journal)

FREE GUIDED MEDITATION SCRIPTS AND DOWNLOADS

http://www.chopra.com/articles/guided-meditations

http://www.innerhealthstudio.com/meditation-scripts.html

MEDITATION PROGRAMS OFFERING PERSONAL MANTRAS

Chopra Center-Primordial Sound Meditation (PSM)
http://www.chopra.com/online-courses/primordial-sound-meditation/on-demand#sm.000011af3bkgbdfkaw6j53wcpiqs6
Maharishi Mahesh-Transcendental Meditation (TM)
http://www.tm.org/

ABOUT THE AUTHOR

Jennifer Millette, LCSW, LMT, E-RYT 200, is an integrative health coach and self-care advocate. Her specialties include stress reduction, burnout prevention and maintaining work-life balance. Her holistic approach helps clients restore energy, vitality and well-being. Jennifer lives, works and plays in the Chicagoland area.